Homeopathy for Headaches: A Doctor's Easy Guide to Prescribing

By Igor Ostrovsky, MD, PhD

Illustrations by Annie Dwyer

Forward by Bhawisha and Shachindra Joshi, MD (Hom)

Contents

Dedication

I dedicate this book to the memory of the late Dr. Nicholai Slupsky (1899–1964), who by virtue of his superb surgical skills and unconventional thinking saved my life when I was a child, and who became the reason I've practiced medicine for the last 40 years, embracing the wisdom of its conventional and unconventional ways.

And to all my mentors of different medical specialties and countries—the United States, Russia, Germany, Switzerland, India, and China—who guided me in the vast ocean of medical knowledge and experience, and who contributed to my current vision of medicine.

Forward

This precise, compact, and useful book offers a clinical approach to one of the most bothersome complaints—headache. It is a complaint that makes everyone—both the sufferer and the helper—impatient.

We have known Dr. Igor Ostrovsky for more than a decade since we first met him in Vermont. His interactions and inputs in our seminars were valuable and clear, just like this book.

Dr. Ostrovsky has touched on the philosophy and modus operandi of homeopathy and homeopaths, a science more popular in India than in the West. His work gives the reader insight into the philosophy and profound benefits of the science.

For a patient, a symptom is just a symptom—but for the homeopath, this symptom has almost an entire personality and various facets to it, from location and sensation to modality and concomitants. This is the depth to which a homeopath explores every symptom.

Dr. Ostrovsky aptly uses this understanding to highlight peculiarities of the remedies, including brief references to their personality types. This is the fundamental basis of the science, making it more holistic and person-specific rather than symptom or pathology-specific. A complete prescription always has lasting results.

We believe this book is an apt tool to help homeopaths make astute prescriptions when it comes to headaches. Pictures and case examples throughout the book help to bring the entire clinical picture to life. Read it to unfold the potential of the magic pill!

—Bhawisha Joshi, MD (Hom) and Shachindra Joshi, MD (Hom)

Introduction

Headaches are ubiquitous. And let's face it. Treating headaches can be a headache.

Doctors of every specialty see patients with persistent headaches who are not satisfied with their treatment results. They are searching for alternative solutions including homeopathy. I have a busy integrative pain management practice in New York, where our approach to treating headaches includes homeopathy as well as neural therapy, trigger point injections, chiropractic treatments, and nutritional and hormonal modifications. We successfully treat many patients with chronic headaches.

After medical school, I spent many years studying at the New York School of Homeopathy and taking courses from world-renowned homeopaths. In my experience, migraine, tension, and cluster headaches all respond well to homeopathy. I wrote this book for doctors who want to start using homeopathy but find it complicated and time-consuming. Drawing from many years of treating patients with headaches, I distilled the vast ocean of homeopathic information to the most essential drops that work for doctors in busy practices.

The book's easily digestible format helps novice homeopaths learn how to treat headaches and lets mature homeopaths organize their knowledge and simplify their choice of remedies. This book offers valuable tips for selecting headache remedies swiftly and effectively. It also opens the door to the world of homeopathy if you are just beginning your journey.

What This Book Is NOT and What It IS

This book is not a quick-fix self-help guide like "5 Easy Steps to Beat Your Headache" or "Everything You Need to Know to Cure a Migraine." Nor does it aspire to be a complete resource for headache remedies. In fact, I left out some popular homeopathic remedies because, over many years of practice, I haven't had a chance to apply them all successfully for headaches.

Rather, this book reflects my humble personal experience in the practical application of knowledge that I acquired from highly respected modern and old-time homeopathic doctors.

Choosing a homeopathic remedy may require a substantial time investment. In this book, I share my ways of choosing remedies that fit the time constraints of a busy medical practice. For ease of prescribing, I bundled the remedies into groups emphasizing their clinical aspects, rather than according to their kingdoms or botanical families.

Homeopathic prescribing is largely based on pattern recognition. The prescriber needs to match the patient's symptoms with a toxicologic picture of the remedy (we will discuss this process in the "Law of Similars" chapter). For visual learners, I've included several vivid illustrations to help enhance your memorization.

Headache Classification, Statistics, & Important Facts

Headaches fall into two categories: primary and secondary. Primary headaches—which include tension, migraine, and cluster headaches—are benign, recurrent headaches with no known underlying cause. Secondary headaches spring from an underlying disease or condition, such as a vascular disorder, tumor, head injury, infection, substance use, or substance withdrawal.

Headache statistics are mind-boggling:

- Lifelong prevalence of headache is 96%, with a female predominance
- Tension headaches constitute the bulk of headaches and affect up to 40–50% of the population (1, 2), while migraine headaches affect 10–14.7% (1, 3)
- Though cluster headaches represent only 0.1 % of the population (1, 4), this translates to a large number of people who suffer from them

Migraine headache is the third most prevalent disorder in the world after tension headaches and cavities of the teeth (5). Migraines occur most commonly between the ages of 25 and 55 years and are three times more common in females (1, 6). This has practical implications for prescribing homeopathic remedies, because many of the remedies that we use to treat headaches are traditionally considered more suitable for females.

Most migraine attacks are unilateral and may be accompanied by visual disturbances; nausea and vomiting; extreme sensitivity to noise, light, touch, or smell; and tingling or numbness in the extremities, face, or other areas.

Despite the fact that it may cause significant disability, migraine remains underdiagnosed and undertreated (6). Many patients prefer to self-medicate and do not seek professional help.

Considered the most painful headaches, cluster headaches are accompanied by unilateral autonomic manifestations such as red eye, swelling around the eye, tearing, drooping eyelid, or stuffy or runny nose.

Tension-type headaches are typically less severe and don't come with visual or sensory impairment (aura), vomiting, or sensitivity to light and noise.

This book will address post-traumatic and sinus headaches, which fall into the category of secondary headaches. However, it will not address secondary headaches due to tumors or aneurysms, as the treatment pathway will drastically differ for these conditions.

1. Rizzoli P, Mullally WJ. Headache. Am J Med. 2018 Jan;131(1):17–24.
2. Loder E, Rizolli P. Tension-type headache. BMJ. 2008 Jan 12; 336(7635):88–92.
3. Burch RC, et al. The prevalence and burden of migraine and severe headache in the United States: updated statistics from government health surveillance studies. Headache. 2015 Jan;55(1):21–34.
4. Wei DY, Khalil M, Goadsby PJ. Managing cluster headache. Pract Neurol. 2019 Dec;19(6):521–528.
5. Steiner TJ, et al. Headache disorders are third cause of disability worldwide. J Headache Pain. 2015;16:58.
6. Robbins MS, Lipton RB. The epidemiology of primary headache disorders. Semin Neurol. 2010;30:107–119.

Causes of Headaches

There are plenty of reasons to have headaches. Headaches may arise from psycho-emotional factors and could even be physical expressions of anxiety, depression, or anger. Patients frequently say that stress causes their headaches, though stress usually falls into the same realm of psycho-emotional factors with underlying emotions of anxiety or fear.

Genetics plays a role in the development of migraine and cluster headaches, but that doesn't help us find the correct homeopathic remedy.

Food sensitivity, in my experience, is a frequent cause of headaches, and it deserves special discussion in a separate chapter (see "Trigger Foods, Food Sensitivity, & Diet") or even a separate book.

Head trauma may be a more frequent cause of headaches than generally assumed. In my practice, we usually rely on a patient's report about the history of their head injury. However, sometimes it's difficult to establish a connection between the head injury and current headache because the traumatic event occurred long ago, there was no loss of consciousness, or there was no diagnosis of concussion at that time. So, we have to do very diligent history-taking.

Sinusitis as a source of headaches may also be overlooked if the aggravation occurred long ago, the patient was treated with antibiotics, and the current symptoms are mild (like postnasal drip, which the patient doesn't consider important). So again, we have to dig deep into the patient's history.

Conventional Treatment Options

The list of conventional pharmacological and surgical treatments for headaches is long and impressive, even in this brief and unquestionably incomplete version:

- NSAIDs (ibuprofen, aspirin)
- Acetaminophen
- Caffeine (Excedrin®)
- Triptans
- Opioids
- Benzodiazepines
- Antiepileptic drugs (carbamazepine, Trileptal®, gabapentin, pregabalin, topiramate)
- Tricyclic antidepressants
- Skeletal muscle relaxants (cyclobenzaprine)
- Corticosteroids
- CGRP inhibitors
- Transcutaneous nerve stimulators
- Occipital nerve block
- Sphenopalatine ganglion neurostimulator
- Sphenopalatine ganglion cryoablation
- Surgery on the trigeminal nerve
- Deep brain stimulation (placing an electrode in the hypothalamus)

Every year, a number of new medications enters the market. Needless to say, they all have unwanted side effects that limit their use. The fast-paced expansion of the list, and the emergence of newer and more aggressive surgical treatments, reflects patients' dissatisfaction and desperation regarding treatment results.

Why Do We Use Homeopathy?

Homeopathic remedies are nontoxic, and there are no side effects because the doses are minuscule. At the beginning of his homeopathic career in the late 1700s, Samuel Hahnemann, a German physician and the father of homeopathy, was using conventional doses of medications and started diluting them to get rid of the side effects while keeping the curative effects. He found that the latter is possible if the remedy is chosen on the principle of simillimum, which I will explain shortly.

Another reason to treat a patient homeopathically is that other treatments didn't work. In fact, patients who tried all possible treatments and didn't get good headache relief constitute most of the cases that we see. These patients often ask if they can try something new like homeopathy, neural therapy, trigger point injections, or nutritional modifications.

The Law of Similars

The basis for homeopathy (and its most important principle) is the Law of Similars. Hahnemann discovered this law, which is often summarized as "like cures like." It means that a substance that brings on symptoms in a healthy person can treat an illness with similar symptoms in a sick person. In fact, the word "homeopathy" means "similar suffering."

To prescribe a correct remedy to a patient, we need to find the simillimum—the remedy whose toxicologic picture matches the patient's symptoms. Most of this book is about just that: how to find the simillimum.

Potencies or Dilutions

It's important to choose the correct potency or dilution for each case. Traditionally, potencies are measured in decimals or centesimals. In the centesimal scale, a substance is diluted successively 100 times its original volume each stage. 6C means that the remedy was diluted six times one hundredfold. 30C means that the remedy was diluted 30 times one hundredfold. 6X or D means that the remedy was diluted six times tenfold. 30X or D means that the remedy was diluted 30 times tenfold.

In the United States, we traditionally use centesimal potencies. Small dilutions, like 6C, are traditionally used to treat physical pathology on the organ or tissue level. Dilutions 200C and higher are more often used to address psycho-emotional issues.

Practical Hints for Successful Prescribing

There is no universal remedy for headaches. To prescribe a homeopathic remedy, it is not enough to know that the patient has headaches. It is not enough even to know that the patient has migraine, cluster, or tension headaches. For a successful prescription, we need to know more about the headache and the patient's particular and peculiar ways of interacting with his or her environment. Typically, the latter is the most decisive piece of information. In other words, we prescribe a homeopathic remedy based on what makes this particular patient different from other patients with headaches.

For example, we look at:

- Localization, lateralization, extension of pain, whether the pain is on the right or the left, where it started and where it extended
- Qualities of pain—Is it sharp, dull, burning, hammering, or pressing?
- Concomitant symptoms like vomiting, photophobia, visual disturbances, and weakness
- What makes pain better or worse; for example, is the pain better when pressing on the painful spot or when using an ice pack, or is it worse when the patient is hungry?
- Etiology of pain—Is the headache due to a head injury or sunstroke that the patient suffered from a few years ago, or due to menopause, gynecological, or gastrointestinal issues?
- Timing and pace of symptom development

Bilateral Headache Remedies

While some remedies are more helpful for left- or right-sided headaches, other remedies treat bilateral headaches, which have no preferential lateralization of pain. Let's start with remedies for bilateral headaches.

If the pain starts in the occiput and then extends forward, I think of two remedies: GELSEMIUM and SILICA or SILICEA. Gelsemium is jasmine and Silicea is quartz or sand.

Headaches treated with Gelsemium characteristically extend from the occiput to the whole head, while headaches treated with Silicea also start in the occiput but extend to the eyes.

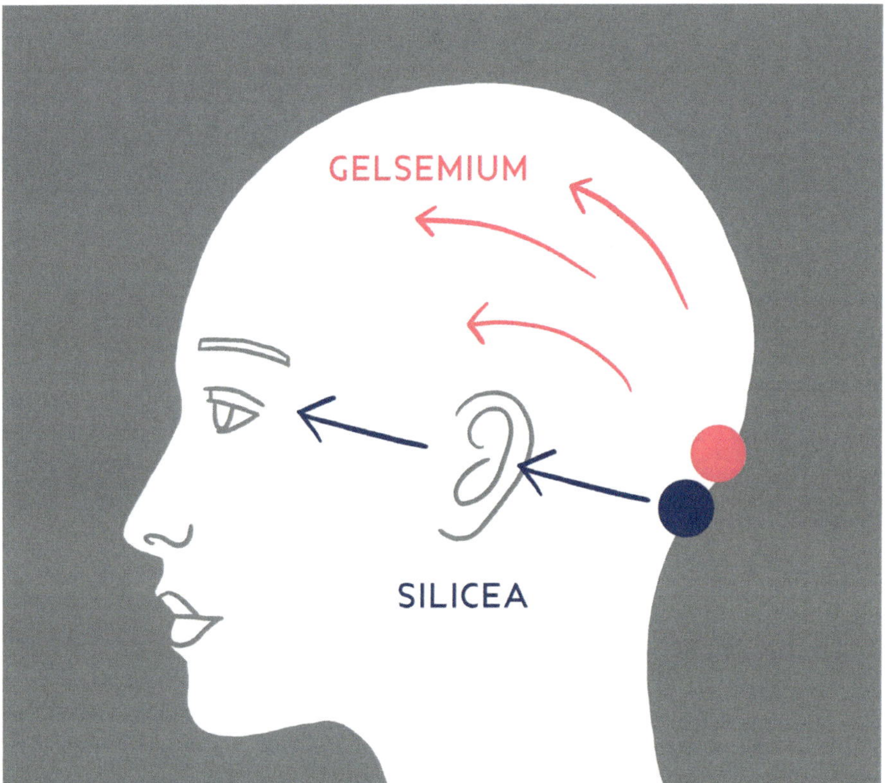

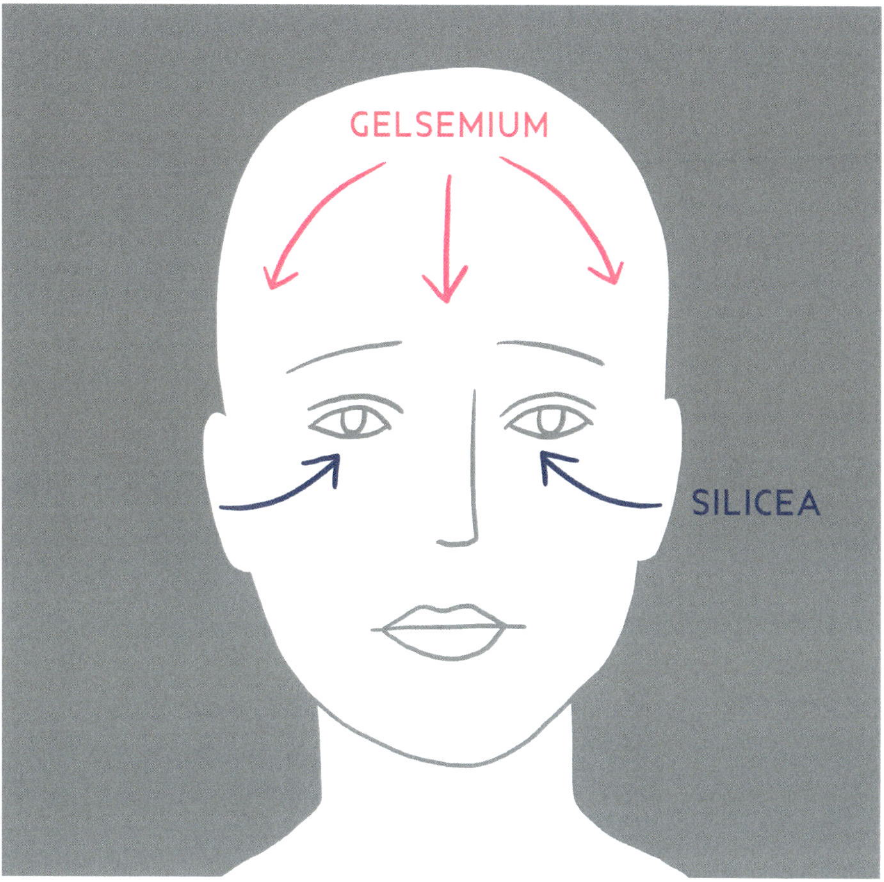

To further distinguish between these two remedies, we can consider other symptoms. Vertigo and weakness are more specific for Gelsemium than for Silicea.

Weakness may manifest in the Gelsemium patient as a sensation of very heavy eyelids. So, if a patient with a headache complains of heavy eyelids, I think of Gelsemium. Yet, they may not say, "my eyelids are heavy"—they may put it differently. One of my patients said, "my eyes are stiff when I have a headache." Upon further questioning I confirmed that this was his expression for heavy eyelids. For him, Gelsemium worked very well. They may also urinate profusely, which, interestingly, improves the headache.

Silicea patients may have severe photophobia. They feel better in a dark room. Other remedies may have this symptom too, but it is very pronounced in Silicea. There is one more remedy, Belladonna (see more about it in "Right-Sided Headaches"), in which the symptom of photophobia is even more pronounced than in Silicea.

Silicea patients are also very chilly, and the cold air makes them feel worse. At night they may even cover their head with a nightcap. These patients are prone to hypothyroidism in a clinical or subclinical form, so they have symptoms like constipation, dry skin, brittle nails, and brittle hair.

Case Study: Silicea
About 10 years ago, I had a 72-year-old female patient who came to see me with Silicea type headaches, but her main complaint was constipation, which was a lifelong problem. The patient knew of her hypothyroidism, but she refused to take any medication for it. Her thyroid-stimulating hormone (TSH) was 54 (normal levels are below 5). Three weeks after I gave her Silicea, her TSH went down to 23, and then in two months to 11, which looked like a miracle to me. Silicea helped her with both symptoms, constipation and migraine headaches. I followed her for a couple of years and she was fine with both symptoms.

The following five additional remedies can also help with headaches when lateralization is not an issue. We choose them on different grounds, and in later chapters I discuss them in greater detail. For now, here is a quick guide:

MERCURIUS SOLUBILIS is made from mercury. Mercury in homeopathic preparations is non-toxic, so you shouldn't worry about it. The most important thing to know about Mercurius headaches is that they may manifest with the sensation "as if a band is around the head."

IRIS is the remedy for headaches that are frequently preceded by a visual aura. But the most important symptom of Iris is vomiting with a very sour taste in the mouth. These patients usually present with gastro-hepatic problems.

PULSATILLA headaches tend to be localized in the forehead. Pulsatilla is also a very important remedy for headaches during menopause. These headaches often find relief with fresh air and cold applications, and they tend to worsen with warmth and sun exposure.

GLONOIN is made from nitroglycerin. We know that nitroglycerin in some patients causes pulsating headaches. They frequently say, "I feel that my head will burst." So, these kinds of headaches are best treated with Glonoin. Additionally, this remedy is also indicated for the treatment of headaches after sunstroke.

STAPHYSAGRIA headaches often start after a confrontation with a partner, and the underlying emotion that triggers the headache is suppressed anger.

Right-Sided Headache Remedies

There are various remedies for right-sided headaches, including those that treat headaches above the right eye.

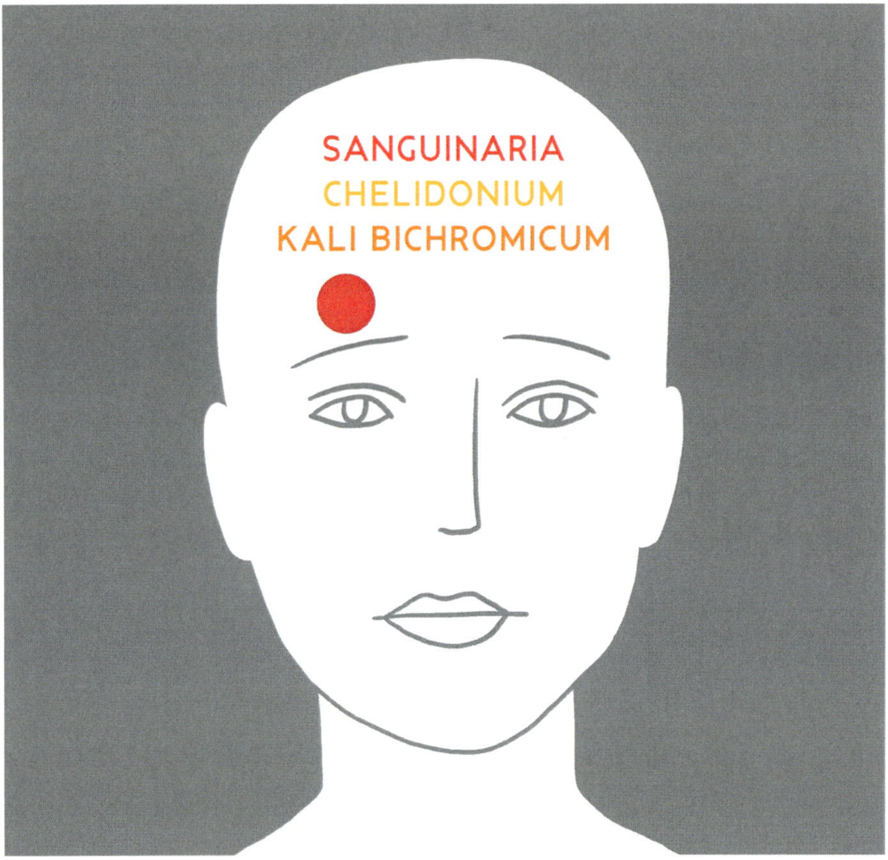

KALI BICHROMICUM is indicated in headaches due to sinusitis. Its characteristic feature is a yellow, sticky nasal discharge where "sticky" is a keyword. Also, this headache improves with a warm application.

SANGUINARIA (bloodroot) headaches may be above the right eye but may also involve the whole right side of the head. The distinguishing feature of Sanguinaria headaches is that vomiting improves the headache.

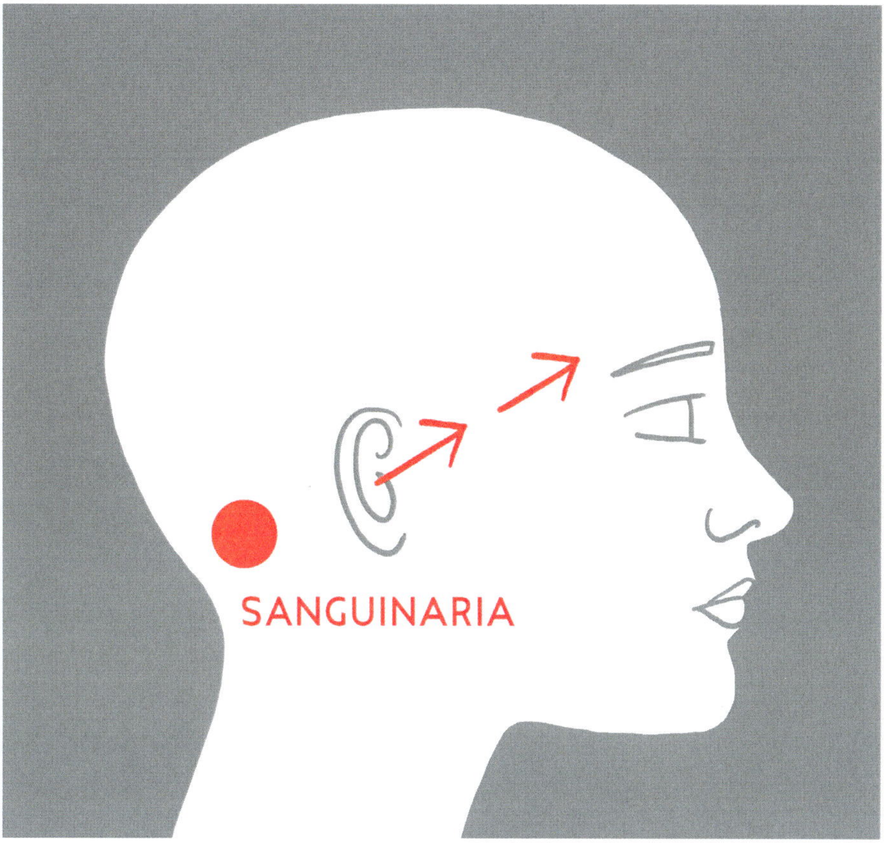

Sanguinaria headaches typically start in the right shoulder or neck and extend above the right eye. The headache's intensity changes gradually during the day. Headaches start in the morning, peak around noon, and decrease by sunset.

CHELIDONIUM (celandines) comes from the same botanical family as Sanguinaria and is indicated in patients with liver and gallbladder disease. In neural therapy and traditional Chinese medicine, the point above the right eye is used to treat gallbladder and liver problems.

Belladonna, Magnesia phosphorica, and Cimicifuga are three more remedies indicated in right-sided headaches.

A characteristic feature of MAGNESIA PHOSPHORICA is that the right-sided headache improves with hard pressure.

MAGNESIA PHOSPHORICA

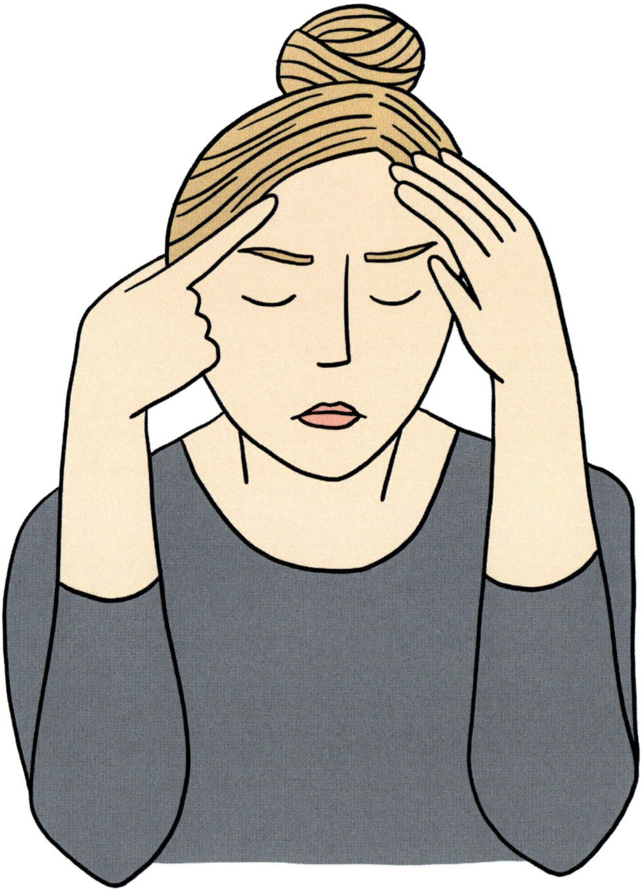

Headaches of CIMICIFUGA RACEMOSA (black cohosh) start in the neck and shoot to the right side of the occiput. Headaches of Cimicifuga may also be in the vertex (top of the head). Cimicifuga is a "female remedy," and headaches of Cimicifuga are worse with menses. Later chapters will discuss this further, including a special chapter on female remedies.

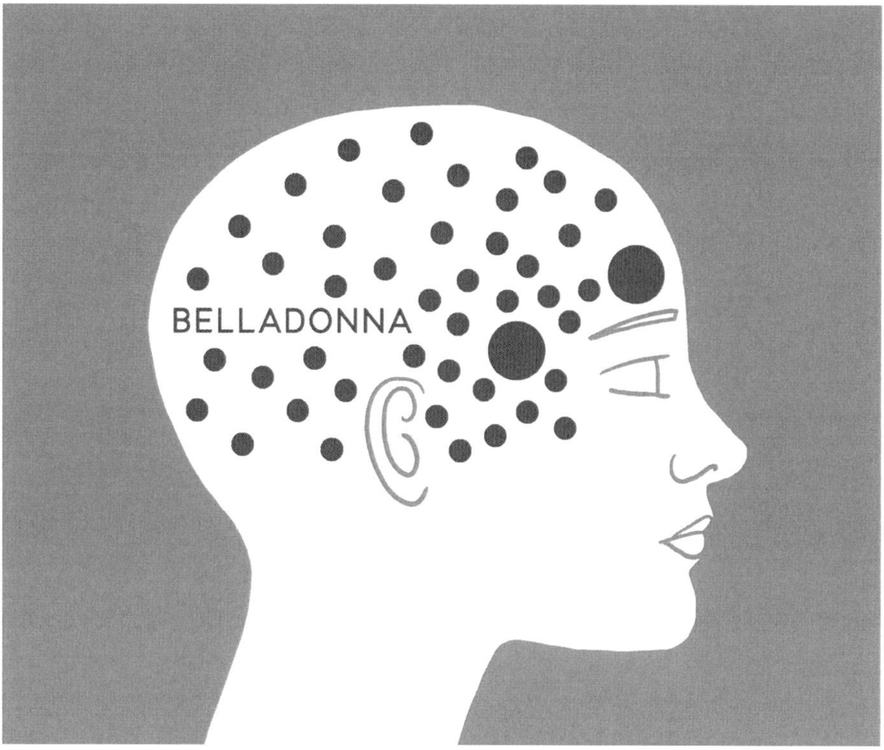

Regarding BELLADONNA headaches, there are three words to remember: violent, sudden, and photophobia.

The full name of the herb is Atropa belladonna (deadly nightshade). It contains the alkaloid atropine, which has anticholinergic effects. So, patients with headaches who can benefit from Belladonna may have symptoms as if they were injected with atropine: tachycardia, dry mouth, dilated pupils, muscle spasms, and twitches of the eyelids or lips. Their severe photophobia results from having very dilated pupils.

Belladonna headaches are the most violent kind. They are frequently located above the right eye or in the right temporal area and may eventually cover the entire head. These extremely intense headaches have a sudden onset and sudden ending, and they may last for hours. Belladonna is frequently indicated in migraine headaches. If you have 10 patients with migraine headaches, two of them will probably benefit from Belladona. These patients describe the pain as throbbing, pulsating, like a knife, like a hammer, or as a sensation of pressure. The head may be hot, and cold applications may improve the headache.

Belladonna type headaches may be aggravated by multiple factors:

- Light (so the patient stays in a dark room)
- Any change of weather
- Heat from the sun
- Warmth
- Sudden jarring

These headaches usually start after 3:00 p.m. and may last through the night. They may also be worse with menses.

Belladonna headaches may improve with:

- Resting in bed
- Staying in a dark room
- Applying hard pressure
- Wearing a tight head bandage

Case Study: Belladonna

A 55-year-old woman came to me complaining of severe migraine headache attacks. Her headaches were right-sided and started around the afternoon, which is typical for Belladonna. They lasted for a few hours and sometimes through the night. She had to stay in a dark room because of severe photophobia. The room had to be not only dark but also isolated, because during these attacks she had such sensitivity that she couldn't even tolerate noise or vibrations of the floor when someone was walking in the room. After the attack ended, she was left completely exhausted and often missed work the next day. This is a typical case of Belladonna. Even if her headaches were not right-sided, I would still have prescribed Belladonna because the intensity of the pain and highly acute symptoms called for this remedy.

Although headaches of both Sanguinaria and Belladonna are right-sided, we can distinguish them because we know that Belladonna is more sudden and intense, while Sanguinaria headaches are gradual. Sanguinaria headaches start in the morning and develop during the day slowly, while Belladonna headaches start suddenly in the afternoon and end suddenly. We also know that both headaches may be accompanied by vomiting, but headaches of Sanguinaria improve with vomiting. Sanguinaria patients may also have an issue with the right shoulder.

Left-Sided Headache Remedies

Left-sided headaches call for different homeopathic treatments, including the following remedies.

SEPIA (cuttlefish) headaches start around the left eye or temple and radiate to the occiput. The most important feature of Sepia is that these headaches improve with intense exercise. So, if I see a patient whose pains get better when she runs a few miles, I think of Sepia. Also, Sepia is what we call a "cold" remedy, and these patients improve with warmth.

Sepia is prescribed most frequently to females. These women are prone to suffer from headaches during their periods. We will discuss Sepia more in the chapter related to female remedies.

SPIGELIA (pinkroot) headaches are typically characterized by left-sided pain in a small spot. The patient can point to the pain spot with her finger. Also, their headaches are up and down with the sun like Sanguinaria headaches. They start in the morning, gradually increase in intensity by noon, and decrease by sunset.

FERRUM METALLICUM (iron) headaches start in the left temple and around the left eye, like Lachesis. The pain is throbbing and hammering, which gets worse after midnight and from violent exertion. They may also have pain in the deltoid muscle of the left shoulder. All pains of Ferrum improve by slowly walking about.

I think of Ferrum metallicum in cases with a history of iron-deficient anemia, orthostasis, vertigo on rising from a chair or from bed, and heavy menstrual or nasal bleeding. Their cheeks flush red easily from emotions and during headaches.

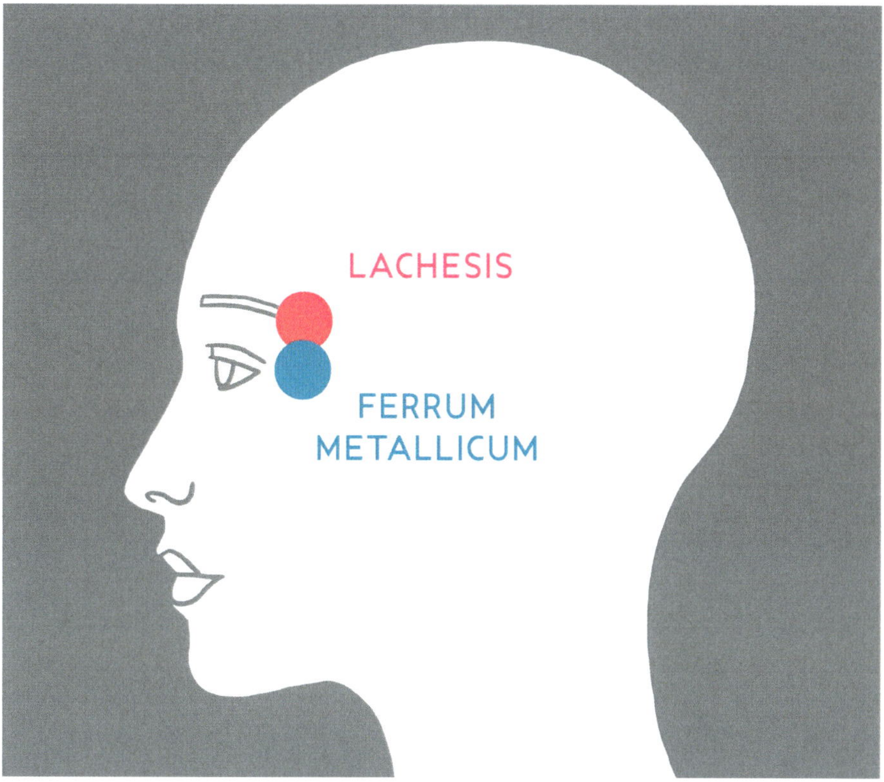

LACHESIS is a remedy made from the venom of a very poisonous snake, Bushmaster, that inhabits Amazon jungles. Headaches of Lachesis are aggravated by warmth and the heat of the sun. Lachesis is a left-sided remedy. These headaches are worse with suppressed menses and better when bleeding starts. Lachesis is a very important remedy for headaches in menopause.

Case Study: Lachesis

Recently, I had a case of a menopausal woman with headaches located in the left temple over the left eye. Her headaches usually started in the morning upon waking, and she felt better in a cold environment. This constellation of symptoms pointed at Lachesis: a menopausal woman (suppressed menses), headaches in the left temple over the left eye, headaches start in the morning upon waking, and the patient prefers a colder environment. So, I prescribed Lachesis, which cleared her headache.

BRYONIA ALBA (white bryony or wild hop) headaches start around the left eye and extend to the occiput. The most important thing to remember about Bryonia is that these headaches get worse with any movement, including movements of the eyes. People with Bryonia headaches feel better when they lie still.

Another important symptom of Bryonia is that these headaches improve with pressure. So, the patient may press on the painful area to relieve the headache, they may lie on the painful side to keep pressure on it, or they may even hold their head with both hands. Bryonia is a "warm remedy," which means these patients tolerate cold better than warmth. Also, they are thirsty and may have dry mouth. And Bryonia patients frequently have gastritis.

Case Study: Bryonia

A woman came to me initially complaining of anxiety and depression, and I couldn't find the right remedy for her until she developed headaches. When she came in with a headache, I saw that it was left-sided and that she was pressing on the painful spot on the left side of the temple. I suspected that it was Bryonia, and when she told me, "My mouth feels so dry!" I had my confirmation. Bryonia cleared her headaches, and it also significantly improved her anxiety and depression. This is how homeopathy works. It doesn't matter if you treat anxiety or headaches—when you prescribe the right remedy, everything gets better.

THUJA OCCIDENTALIS (northern white cedar or eastern white cedar) patients may also have headaches extending from the left eye to the occiput. An interesting feature of Thuja headaches is that they feel better when bending the head forward and worse when bending the head back. At two times of the day, the headache may be worse—three o'clock in the morning and three o'clock in the afternoon. Thuja may also experience other types of headaches—as if the head is squeezed in a vice, or like a nail in the left temple or vertex.

But it is a challenge to prescribe Thuja based on headache symptoms alone. Typically, you have to look at the whole history of the patient. They tend to have sexually transmitted diseases, cystitis, urethritis, condylomas, warts, and periodontal disease. Thuja is a "cold remedy," which means that the patient feels better in a warm environment. If I suspect a case of Thuja, I also check to see if the headaches started after a vaccination of any sort, because Thuja is one of the main remedies for side effects from vaccinations.

Let's take a moment to summarize left-sided headache remedies. Headaches of Lachesis and Ferrum metallicum are fixed in the left temple around the left eye.

Headaches of Sepia, Bryonia, and Thuja start in the area of the left eye and extend to the left side of the occiput. Spigelia headaches start on the left side of the occiput and extend to the left eye. But keep in mind that the patient actually may feel pain in both areas—in the occiput and in the eye—so it is very important to ask about the sequence of events, including where the pain started and where it settled.

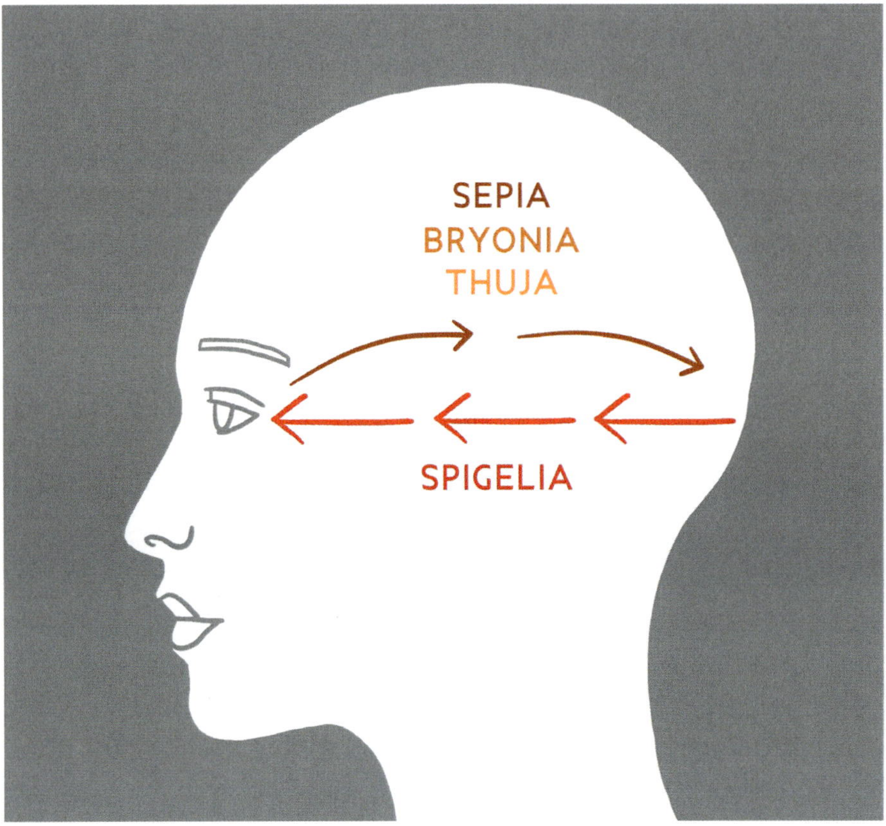
SEPIA
BRYONIA
THUJA
SPIGELIA

Remedies for Headaches in the Vertex

When a Thuja patient has pain in the vertex, it's more likely to be felt as a nail in the vertex, and the patient may also report a similar headache in the left temple.

Cimicifuga is a female remedy. Headaches of Cimicifuga may feel as if they are pressing the vertex upward.

Patients may also report strange sensations in the skull, as if "the skull is open" or as if "wind is blowing in the brain." When a patient reports unusual sensations in the brain, I think of Cimicifuga because due to different backgrounds, people have different ways of expressing their experiences. Headaches of Cimicifuga are frequently aggravated by menses, as every symptom of Cimicifuga is aggravated by menses. These patients also tend to have rheumatic issues.

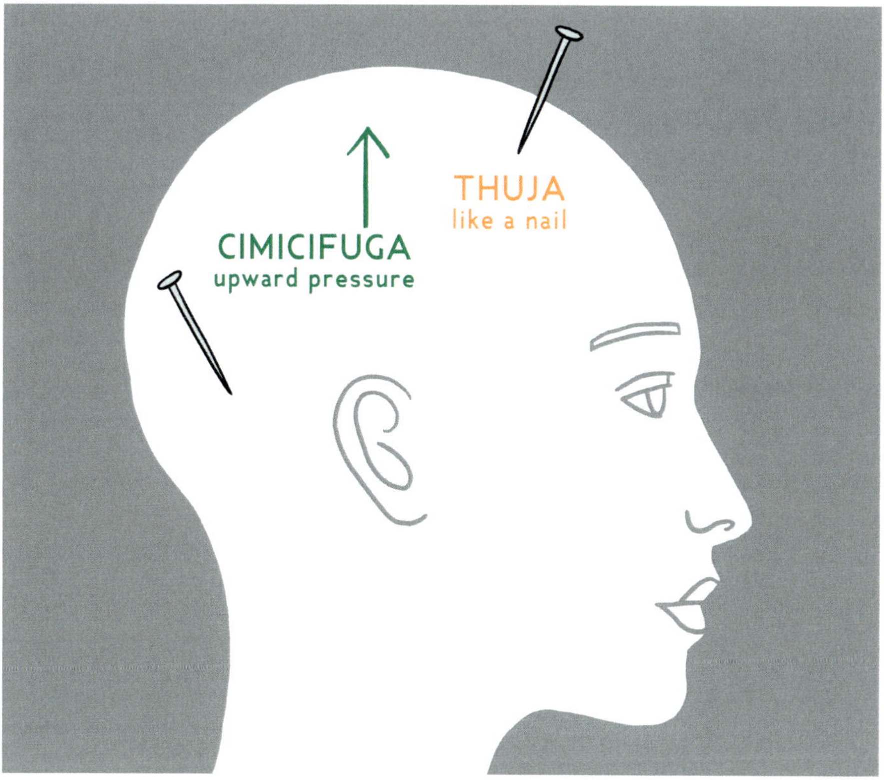

Heat in the Vertex

When a headache in the vertex brings a sensation of heat, I think of two remedies: Lachesis and Sulphur.

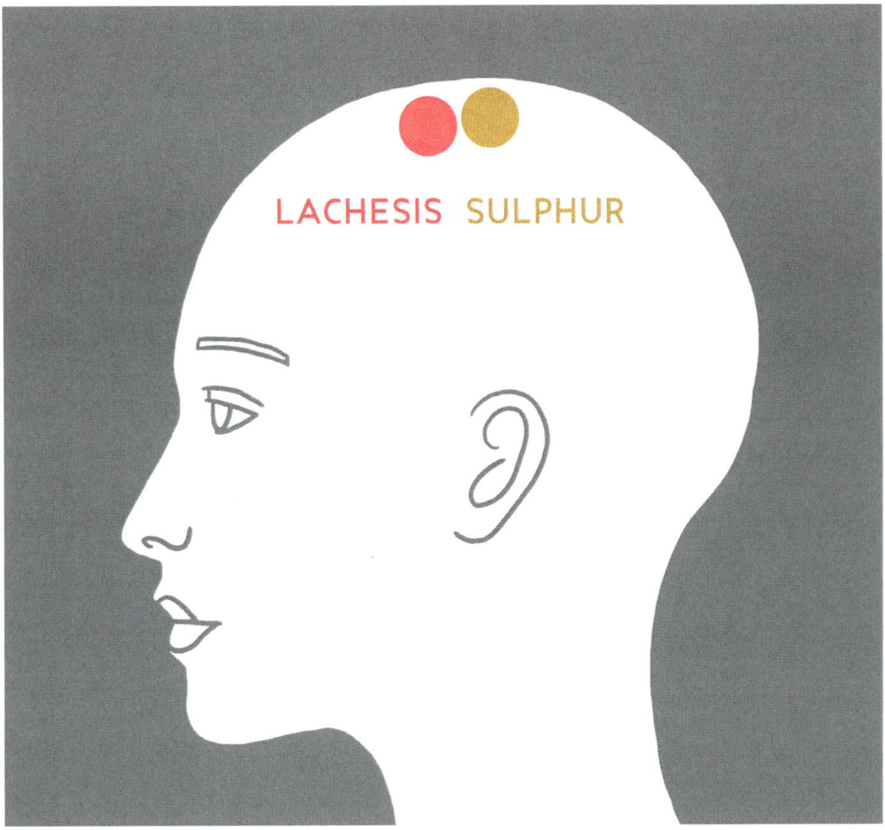

Lachesis is also a female remedy, which we will discuss further in the "Female Remedies" chapter. Lachesis headaches are worse before menses and better when bleeding starts. These patients don't tolerate tight clothing around the neck, and their headaches start when they wake up.

Sulphur patients feel better with cold applications. They may experience the sensation of heat not only in the vertex but also in the forehead. Sulphur patients may develop headaches after suppressed eruptions on the skin. So, if the patient has a history of suppressed eruptions, it is a good idea to start treating them with Sulphur. Be aware that while headaches may improve, the eruptions in the skin may come back. This is a normal outward direction of healing.

Both Lachesis and Sulphur headaches are aggravated by heat and sun. A few years ago, I had a patient who complained of heat in the vertex, for which he applied an ice pack. I found that, a couple of months prior to developing headaches, he had a history of suppressed eruptions. Sulphur successfully cleared his headaches.

Occipital Headache Remedies

Now, let's move on to occipital headaches, where the pain is felt in the back of the head. For the most part, this will be a recap of several remedies that we've already covered.

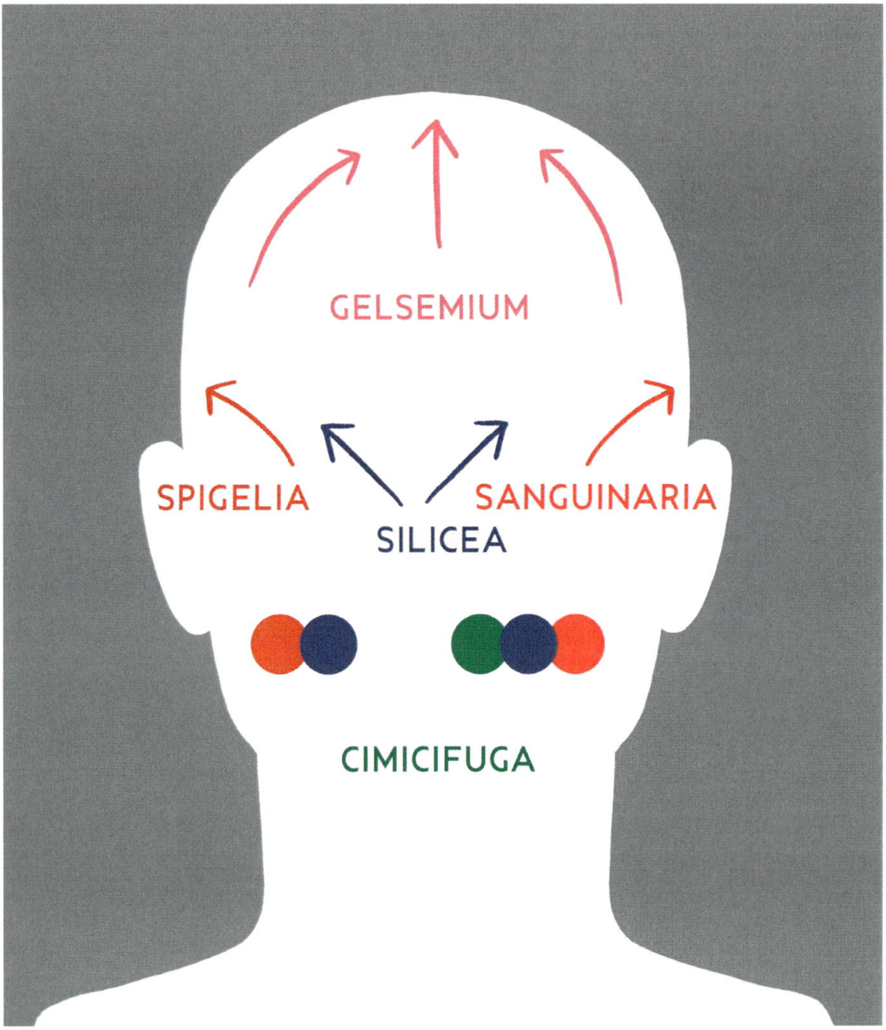

First, a few points to keep in mind:

- Cimicifuga occipital headaches usually feel like a nail in the right side of the occiput. The pain shoots from the neck to the right side of the occiput. It's important to remember that with Cimicifuga, menses aggravates the headache.

- Silicea headaches start in the occiput and extend to the eyes.
- Gelsemium headaches start in the occiput and extend to the whole head.
- Sanguinaria headaches start in the occiput and extend above the right eye.
- Spigelia headaches start in the occiput, extend forward, and stay above the left eye.
- Sepia, Thuja, and Bryonia headaches start around the left eye and extend back to the occiput.

Case Study: Spigelia

A few years ago, I had a patient who complained of headaches around her left eye. When she entered my office, she was pressing her finger on the painful spot. She also told me that she felt a connection between this spot and another area on the left side of the occiput. So, I had to differentiate between Bryonia and Spigelia because she felt pain around her left eye, and pressure helped to alleviate the pain. I determined that this was a case of Spigelia, and this example shows the thought process that I have in mind when choosing a remedy. Of course, there was another sign that confirmed Spigelia—the pain was in a small spot that the patient could point to with her finger.

NATRUM SULPHURICUM and ARNICA MONTANA are two remedies discussed in the section "Post-traumatic Headaches." Both are used to treat occipital headaches.

Arnica patients may complain of headaches in the occiput when the head touches the pillow. In fact, both the pillow and the entire bed feel hard to Arnica patients. This is part of a major issue with Arnica—these patients are very sensitive to touch.

Distribution & Qualities of Pain

Now, let's find out how to prescribe a homeopathic remedy based on the distribution and qualities of the headache.

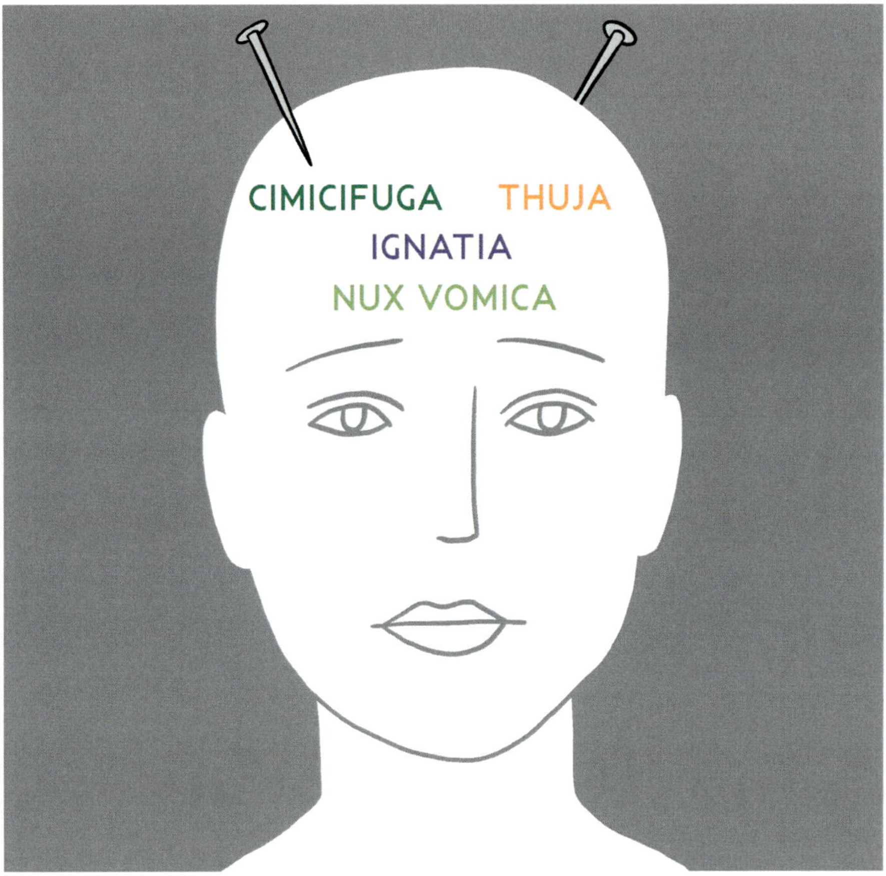

Headaches Like a Nail
When a patient complains of headaches that feel like a nail, I think of four remedies, two of which we've already covered.

If a Cimicifuga patient has a headache like a nail, they usually feel it in the occiput. The pain comes from the neck and feels like a nail in the back of the head.

If a Thuja patient has a headache like a nail, it's often localized in the left temple or in the vertex.

Two additional remedies for this type of headache include IGNATIA AMARA and NUX VOMICA, both made from plants containing strychnine.

Nux vomica patients may have a headache like a nail, but the quality of the headache doesn't matter. We choose Nux vomica on different grounds. These patients are workaholics who abuse coffee, tobacco, and alcohol as stimulants to keep themselves running. They have a type A personality and may be irritable or angry. Their headaches are worse in the morning, and they are very sensitive patients, aggravated by mental exertion, anger, noise, odors, and touch. Their digestive tract is very sensitive as well, and they're prone to indigestion.

Nux vomica happens to be my favorite remedy for hangover headaches. It can also be used for the early stages of liver cirrhosis, such as fatty liver.

Pain like a nail is also characteristic of Ignatia, whether it is pain in the head or pain in other parts of the body. I think of Ignatia when the underlying emotion is grief—for example, grief for a lost loved one. The patient may weep, but she will keep her grief to herself and she is not looking to be consoled.

Headaches Like a Band Around the Head

If the headache feels like a band around the head, I think of three remedies: Mercurius, Gelsemium, and Sanguinaria.

Mercurius patients feel as if they're wearing a helmet or tight hat around the head. Gelsemium patients may have a similar feeling because Gelsemium headaches start in the occiput and radiate through the temples to the whole head. So, they may describe the pain as a band around the head. And Sanguinaria patients may have the feeling of a band that goes halfway around on the right side—because this right-sided headache starts in the occiput and extends through the temple to the front of the head, above the right eye.

Female Remedies

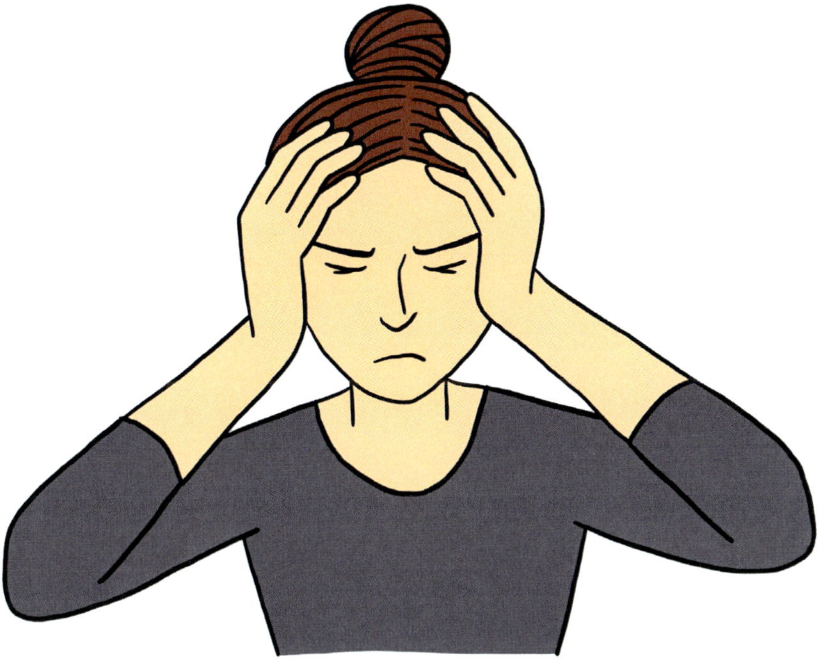

Four remedies—Sepia, Pulsatilla, Cimicifuga, and Lachesis—have a strong propensity to act on the female reproductive organs. These remedies are prescribed to females more frequently than to males, and these patients are prone to menstrual disorders and issues around menopause. Their headaches worsen around menses and improve with fresh air.

Pulsatilla and Lachesis are warm remedies. These patients prefer a colder environment and don't like being in a warm environment. On the other hand, Sepia and Cimicifuga are cold remedies. These individuals prefer a warm environment and don't like being in a cold environment.

Pulsatilla, Sepia, and Cimicifuga patients have a tendency to weep. They may weep during the consultation as they are talking about their headaches. Sepia and Cimicifuga patients are irritable with a sense of anger. So, if I see an angry, weeping patient, I think of Sepia and Cimicifuga. Even if a Pulsatilla patient is irritable, she is not angry.

Let's take a closer look at each of these four female remedies:

Sepia headaches originate over the left eye and radiate into the occiput. Even more important, they improve with intense exercise. So, if a patient tells me that her headaches or other symptoms feel better when she runs a few miles, I think of Sepia. Interestingly, these patients are prone to a "bearing down" feeling in the uterus or a sensation of a lump or ball in the pelvis because they have a predisposition to uterine prolapse. They may have these sensations even if they have not yet been diagnosed with uterine prolapse. Sepia is a cold remedy, so these patients feel better with warmth. They may also be weepy and irritable.

Pulsatilla is a remedy that I frequently prescribe for headaches during menopause. These headaches are usually around the forehead, above the eyes, and they're worse in the evening and at night. A very important symptom is that these headaches change location. Today the pain may be in one place; tomorrow it will be in another place. They have a tendency for light menses or even amenorrhea. Even if a Pulsatilla patient is chilly, they will feel worse with warmth and they'll open windows even in wintertime to let the air in. Pulsatilla patients tend to be weepy. Another characteristic is that they are thirstless.

Cimicifuga headaches are worse with menses. These patients have headaches in the vertex, pressing upwards. They may have headaches in the right side of the occiput, and they may have strange sensations in the skull, as if "the skull is open" or "a wind is blowing in the brain." Though they feel better with fresh air and like to be outside, these patients are aggravated by cold. They're prone to weepiness and irritability, and they tend to have rheumatic issues—which is often an important confirmation sign. They're also prone to depression. So, if their headache is aggravated during menses, and the patient is prone to depression, I think of Cimicifuga.

With Lachesis, it's important to remember that these headaches are worse before menses, when the flow is suppressed. Menopause is another situation where flow is suppressed. All symptoms, including headaches, are better when menses start. Lachesis patients may have headaches in the left temple around the left eye, and their headaches are worse in the morning upon waking up. A peculiar issue for Lachesis patients is tremendous sensitivity in the area of the neck. They are so sensitive to touch that they do not tolerate tight clothing around the neck. Warmth and sun make them feel worse.

In a psychological aspect, these patients may be sexual, jealous, critical, or suspicious. If they suppress their sexuality, they may be religious and loquacious. So, anytime I see a patient who is talking a lot, I think first of Lachesis.

For Better or Worse

In this chapter, we'll discuss how to choose remedies based on what makes a headache better or worse.

If a tight bandage helps to relieve headaches, I think of Belladonna, Gelsemium, Silicea, and Magnesia phosphorica.

BELLADONNA
GELSEMIUM
SILICEA
MAGNESIA PHOSPHORICA

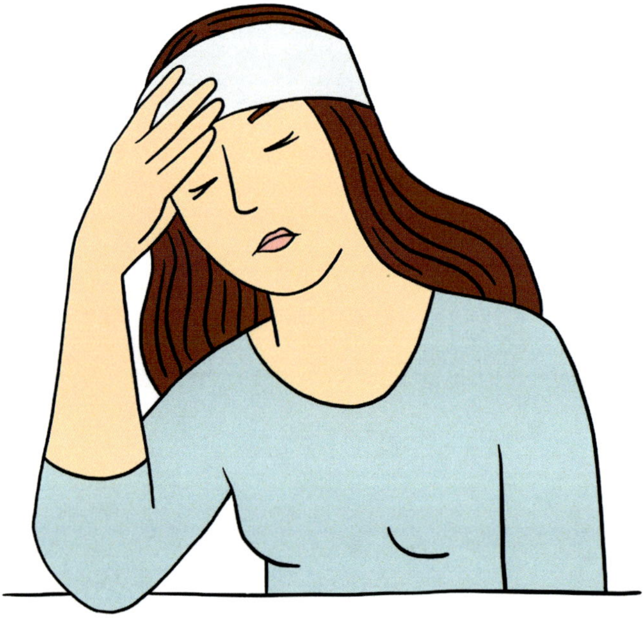

Sanguinaria headaches are better with massage, and Bryonia headaches are better with hard pressure yet worse with light touch.

Belladonna, Arnica, and Lachesis are worse with touch, and Bryonia is worse with light touch and better with hard pressure.

Another remedy not discussed yet is MEZEREUM. For these patients, the head is so sensitive to light touch that they may have pain even when combing their hair. Mezereum patients usually have eruptions on the head.

Warm Remedies

Sanguinaria, Bryonia, Pulsatilla, Natrum sulphuricum, Sulphur, and Lachesis are warm remedies. These patients get worse with warmth and prefer a colder environment.

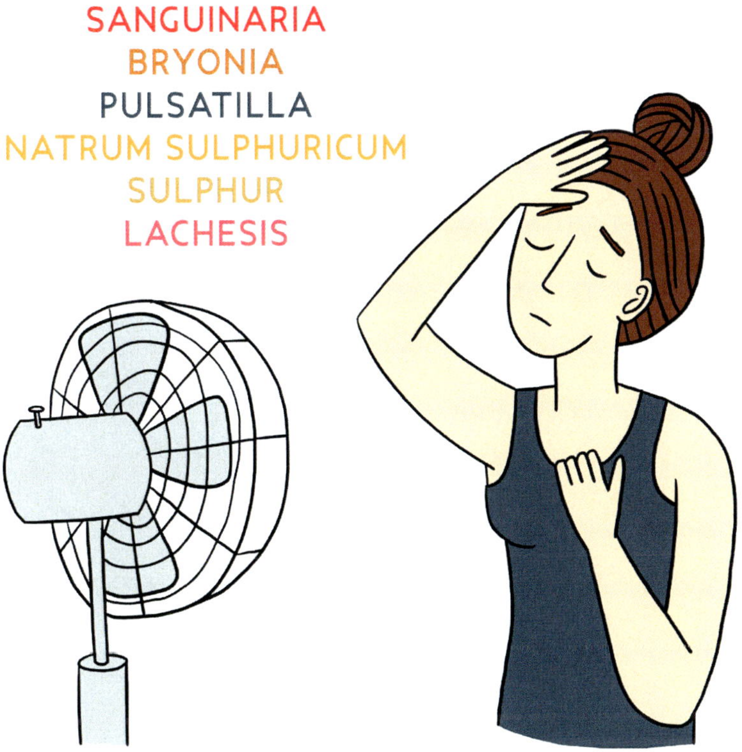

If headaches improve with cold applications, I think of Belladonna, Sulphur, Pulsatilla, and Lachesis.

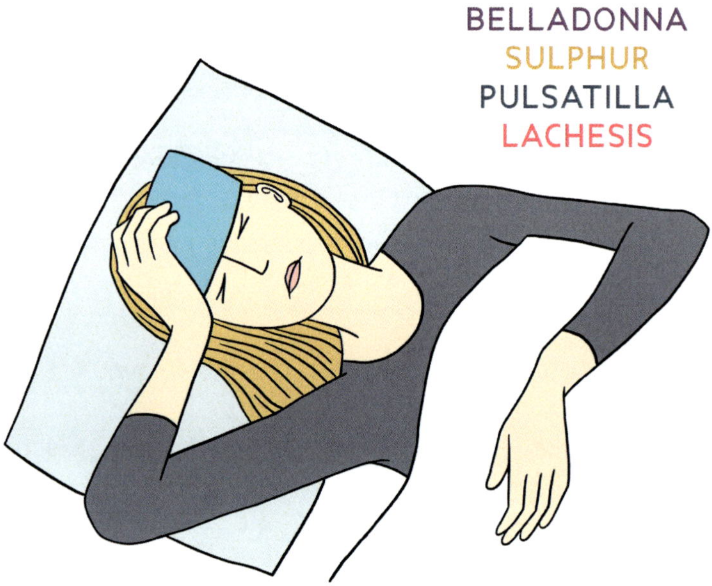

Cold Remedies

Silicea, Thuja, and Sepia are cold remedies. The cold aggravates these patients, and they prefer a warm environment.

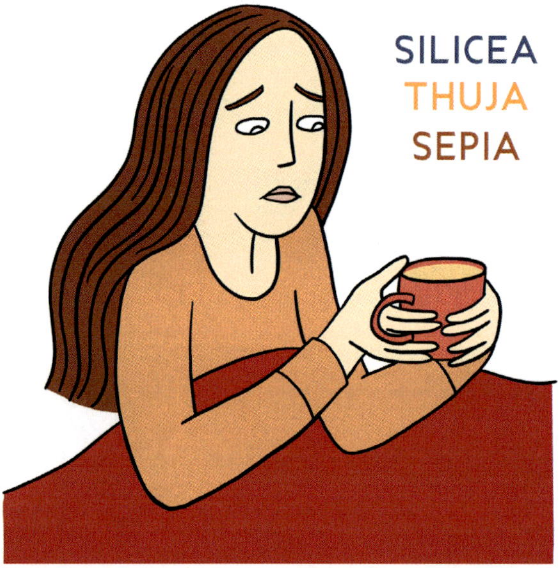

If a patient's headache is relieved by covering the head—for example, with a nightcap—I think of Silicea. Silicea happens to be one of the chilliest remedies.

SILICEA

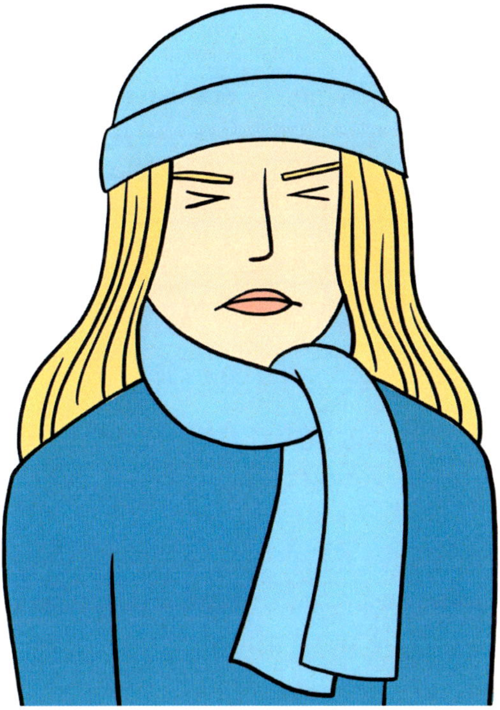

Weather & Headaches

If a patient tells me that his headaches get worse with a change of weather, I listen very carefully because it helps me to choose the remedy.

Belladonna, Sulphur, Lachesis, and Glonoin headaches are aggravated by sun exposure. Belladonna headaches may get worse with drafts of cold air and a wet head. Some of these patients may get a headache when they go outside after a shower or bath, without having dried their head completely.

Any symptom of Natrum sulphuricum, including headaches, gets worse with humid weather. Once I was choosing between Natrum sulphuricum and Arnica for headaches, and I gave preference to Natrum sulphuricum because the patient reported to me that his symptoms are worse in wet weather.

RHUS TOXICODENDRON (poison ivy) headaches are aggravated by wet and cold weather. Headaches of Rhus toxicodendron are usually accompanied by neck pain and stiffness. All Rhus symptoms, including headaches, are better with motion (like Ferrum) and worse with rest.

Occasionally, I see patients whose headaches are better at the seashore. In these cases, I think of MEDORRHINUM. (Although not discussed at length in this book, Medorrhinum falls into a special group called nosodes and may figure into a future book about the treatment of rheumatic conditions.) These patients usually specify that their headaches' improvement is not about being on vacation in a stress-free environment, but about being close to the seashore. In my experience, they readily report this symptom without targeted questioning because they consider it strange and unusual.

Prescribing Based on Concomitant Symptoms

Let's discuss how to prescribe remedies based on concomitant symptoms.

Weekend Headaches
When I see a patient who has headaches on the weekends, I think of IRIS VERSICOLOR (northern blue flag). Weekend headaches are also called relaxation headaches. We don't know why they happen, but some speculate that they arise due to an abuse of caffeine and sugar during weekdays and a lack of those on weekends. These are hard-working people and their symptoms get better when they work (homeopaths use the term "occupation ameliorates"). In a way, this is reminiscent of Nux vomica, but Nux vomica headaches are not specific to weekends. Iris headaches are localized in a small spot, like Kali bichromicum and Spigelia.

Hunger Headaches
I think of LYCOPODIUM when a patient tells me that she has headaches when she misses her meals.

Headaches with Vomiting
When headaches are accompanied by vomiting, I think of three remedies: Sanguinaria, Belladonna, and Iris.

Sanguinaria headaches improve with vomiting. Belladonna and Iris headaches do not improve with vomiting.

Iris vomiting has a peculiar symptom—it leaves a very sour taste in the mouth. As one old-master homeopath once said, "Everything in the stomach turns into vinegar." The vomitus is stringy, and they may have a burning sensation in the stomach. These are usually patients with gastro-hepatic issues.

SANGUINARIA

vomiting improves headache

BELLADONNA

vomiting does not improve headache

IRIS

vomiting does not improve headache;
very sour taste

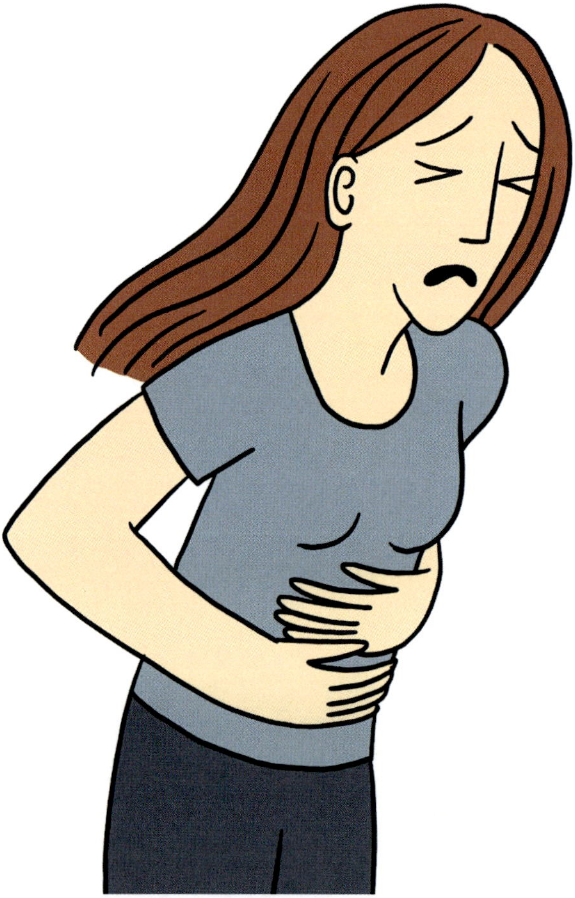

Headaches with Weakness

If a headache is accompanied by weakness, I think of Gelsemium, especially if the patient reports heaviness of the eyelids. Yet they may use different words to describe this sensation. One of my patients said, "I have stiffness of my eyes when I have a headache," while another patient told me, "I have difficulty seeing when I have a headache." In the latter case, it took me a few minutes of questioning to understand that she meant heaviness of the eyelids. That's why she had difficulty seeing.

Prescribing Based on Headache Etiology

To choose a homeopathic remedy based on the headache's etiology, look for issues like these in the patient's current or past experience:

- **Vaccinations**. If the patient's headaches started after a vaccination of any sort, consider Silicea and Thuja as remedies.
- **Menopause and perimenopause**. If a woman's headaches started in the perimenopausal period, I think of Pulsatilla, Sepia, and Lachesis.
- **Childbirth**. If a woman's headaches started after childbirth, possible remedies include Sepia, Pulsatilla, and Cimicifuga.
- **Suppressed eruptions**. If the patient's headache started after suppressed eruptions, a suitable remedy is Sulphur.
- **Sunstroke**. If their headaches started after sunstroke, consider Belladonna, Lachesis, Sulphur, and Glonoin.
- **Trauma**. For post-traumatic headaches, I most frequently choose between Arnica and Natrum sulphuricum. The following section explores this choice in greater detail.

HEADACHES IN MENOPAUSE

PULSATILLA
SEPIA
LACHESIS

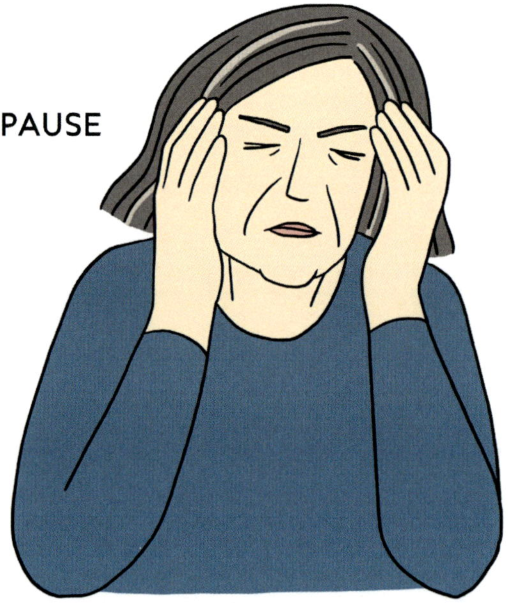

Post-traumatic Headaches

With any patient experiencing headache, I check to see if his headache could have been caused by a traumatic event, either recently or in the past. Trauma of the head may be responsible for a patient's symptoms for years after the injury. So, the important thing is to find out if there was a traumatic event before the headaches started. And the problem that we frequently encounter is that in many cases, patients don't remember the traumatic event. Either they were small kids at the time of trauma, their parents didn't tell them, their parents were not present during the event, or perhaps they didn't consider the event to be traumatic because there was no diagnosed brain concussion.

Case Study: Natrum sulphuricum

I once treated a doctor's son, a 16-year-old boy, who suffered severe daily headaches for six years. He was on daily ibuprofen. When I asked about injury, the parents said that none had occurred. Finally, I asked if the boy had engaged in any sports before the age of 10, and I found out that he was a trampoline jumper from age five to nine. I asked, "Why did he quit jumping at the age of 9?" And the answer surprised me: "My son didn't want to keep hitting his head." To me, this was an obvious case of multiple head injuries, which led to headaches that started one year after the traumatic events. The boy's parents did not consider the possibility of trauma because there was no diagnosis of brain concussion. I gave him Natrum sulphuricum and his headaches resolved.

For post-traumatic headaches, I usually choose between Arnica and Natrum sulphuricum. In the case study above, I gave the patient Natrum sulphuricum because he preferred being in a cold environment and Natrum sulphuricum is a warm remedy.

ARNICA
NATRUM SULPHURICUM

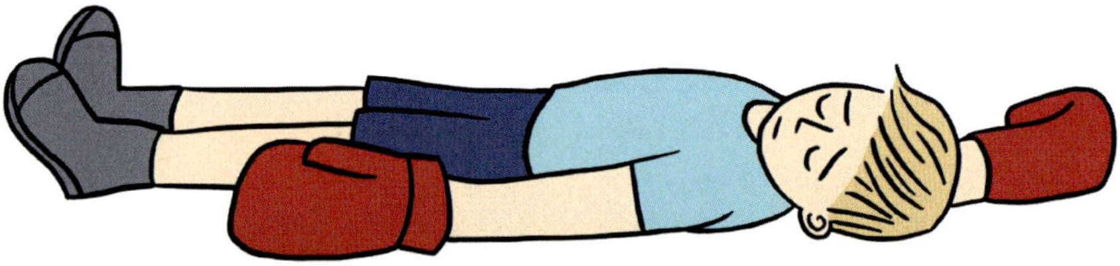

Arnica is the number one remedy for post-traumatic headaches because it is indicated in cases when there was an extravasation of blood, and there is an extravasation of blood in any case of trauma. So, we give Arnica when there was a brain concussion because there are microvascular injuries. We also prescribe Arnica when there was a subdural hematoma or epidural hematoma. Arnica may be given in acute cases and in chronic cases, while Natrum sulphuricum is mostly given in chronic cases of headaches.

I also consider Natrum sulphuricum when there was a significant personality change or physical change in a patient after the trauma. For example, his relatives may say he was a different person before the injury. In general, you may start a case of post-traumatic headache with Arnica and then switch to Natrum sulphuricum if some of the symptoms remain.

Also, keep in mind that head trauma can happen during birth. Any time I see a patient whose headaches started early in life, I consider this possibility.

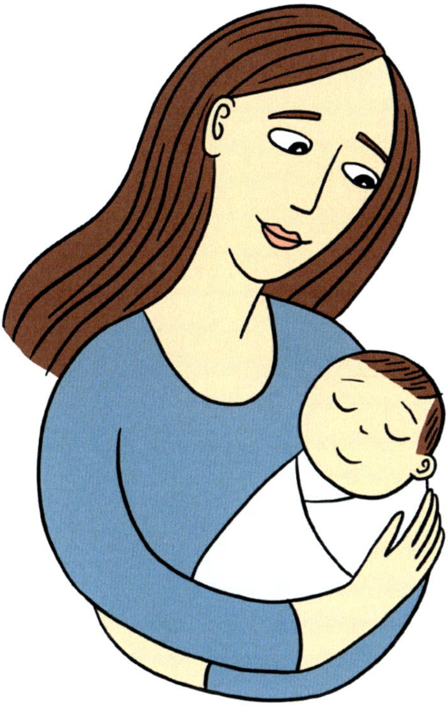

Case Study: Arnica & Natrum sulphuricum

A few years ago, a young woman came to see me who had suffered a serious head injury in a motor vehicle accident two years before. She developed an epidural hematoma that required surgical intervention, and then she developed epileptic seizures and bad headaches. She stopped taking anti-seizure medications because, as she said, "they didn't help anyway." I started treating her with Arnica, which helped with the seizures and decreased her headaches. Later I added Natrum sulphuricum, which cleared her headaches completely.

Surgery is another source of trauma that, ad minimum, produces local damage to blood vessels and tissues, generates fluid shifts, and may cause scarring and leave a psycho-emotional impact. Ad maximum, this trauma can generate lasting symptoms in local and even remote areas of the body. In homeopathy, as well as in neural therapy, this phenomenon is well recognized, and we pay special attention to areas of surgical trauma, even if it happened many years ago. Surgery on the head or face, especially in the area of the nose, in some cases may generate post-traumatic headaches and symptoms in distant parts of the body.

Case Study: Trauma from Surgery

I had a case of a 32-year-old man who came to me complaining of left-sided sciatica and meralgia paresthetica-type numbness in the left thigh. I also learned that he had right-sided temporal headaches, partial hearing loss, and tinnitus. All his symptoms started approximately four years ago, and he denied any head trauma. But I found out that a couple of months prior to the start of his symptoms, he had surgery for nasal polyps and a deviated nasal septum. He thought something had gone wrong during surgery because he never felt well after that. But his ENT doctor couldn't find the cause of his partial hearing loss, and all tests were negative. So, the symptoms were considered unrelated to surgery. Despite that, I treated him as a case of head trauma. I gave him Natrum sulphuricum and it helped to clear his symptoms completely, including the sciatica and numbness in the left thigh. The reason I chose Natrum sulphuricum in this case is that the patient's life changed dramatically after the surgery. He said: "I'm a different person now. I have to adjust my activities to my abilities, to what I can do and what I cannot do." This is a clear indication for Natrum sulphuricum. Another reason I chose Natrum sulphuricum was that he didn't tolerate warmth and preferred a cold environment.

Headaches in School Children

When school children have headaches, I consider CALCAREA PHOSPHORICA for the most part, and occasionally MAGNESIA PHOSPHORICA.

CALCAREA PHOSPHORICA
MAGNESIA PHOSPHORICA

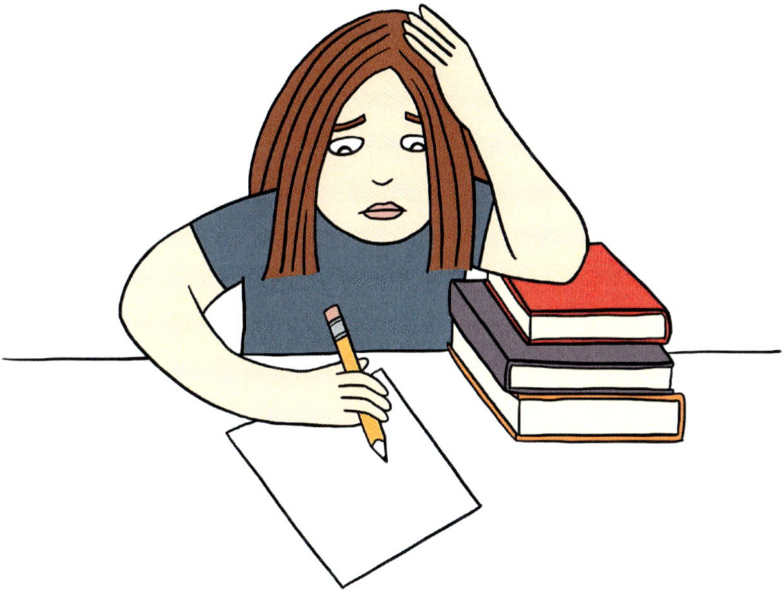

Calcarea phosphorica patients feel worse after mental effort. In advanced cases they may not tolerate physical effort either. In general, they have low vitality and they fatigue easily.

The brain is our most energy-consuming organ. In children, the brain constitutes less than 3% of body weight, yet it consumes more than 20% of the energy produced by the body at rest, and up to 40% during intense mental work. A rapid growth spurt in teenagers may limit the availability of energy to the brain, leading to difficulties in sustaining intense mental effort—and perhaps resulting in headaches. Chemically, Calcarea phosphorica consists mostly of calcium phosphate, which is the main building material for teenagers' rapidly growing bones. This is the easy way to remember that we use Calcarea phosphorica for headaches in school children. Calcarea phosphorica patients may also have issues with the spine. And Calcarea phosphorica is one of the main remedies for children with scoliosis.

Calcarea phosphorica is a cold remedy, meaning that these patients feel worse in cold and wet weather. It's also important to remember that headaches of Calcarea phosphorica usually start in the morning upon waking (like Lachesis).

I think of Magnesia phosphorica in school children if the headache is right-sided, intense and sudden, and improves with hard pressure. Magnesia phosphorica is also one of the main remedies for muscle spasms.

Case Study: Calcarea phosphorica

Older patients with headaches can also benefit sometimes from Calcarea phosphorica. One such patient of mine was a 48-year-old woman and mother of four, who complained of headaches approximately three times a month for many years. Her husband was the head of a pharmaceutical company, so she was able to try different conventional medications, which unfortunately didn't help. When I examined her, I found three important pieces of information: Her headaches had started at age 10, she was easily fatigued, and her headaches were aggravated by intense physical exercise.

We know that Calcarea carbonica (a remedy that we did not discuss in this book) is aggravated by intense physical exercise, while Calcarea phosphorica gets worse with intense mental efforts. Yet, I gave this patient Calcarea phosphorica because her headaches started at age 10, and because in advanced cases, Calcarea phosphorica may also be aggravated by intense physical effort. The remedy successfully cleared her headaches.

STAPHYSAGRIA

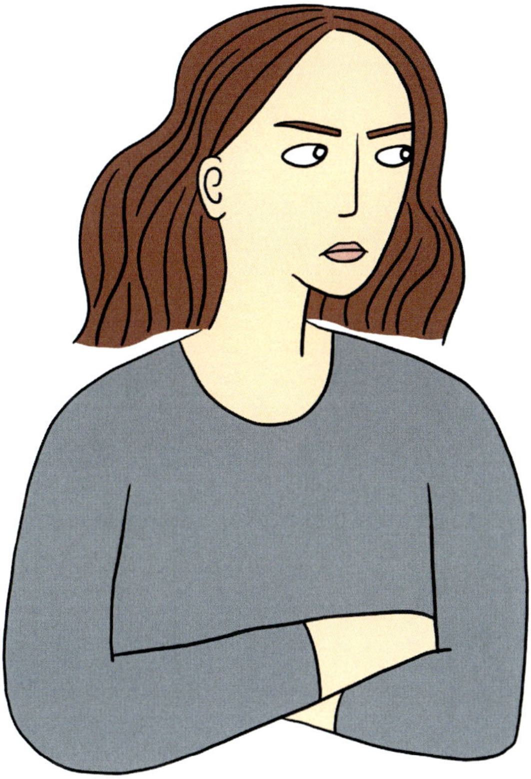

Headaches from Suppressed Anger

In headache cases where the underlying emotion is suppressed anger, I think of Staphysagria. Staphysagria patients usually develop headaches after a confrontation with their partner, when they have to accept the terms of the partner against their will. These patients are kind and soft. They don't revolt and they channel their anger into the physical plane. They may develop headaches, psoriasis, and sties. Staphysagria has a strong connection with sexuality. Women may develop cystitis, while men can develop prostate enlargement, epididymitis, or impotence. And this impotence is of a peculiar nature because they are impotent with their wives with whom they have arguments, but not with other women.

Pace & Timing of Headaches

Now let's look at how the pace and timing of a headache may help us to choose the remedy. Here's a quick guide to prescribing with these factors in mind:

- Belladonna and Magnesia phosphorica headaches start and end suddenly.
- Spigelia and Sanguinaria headaches start in the morning with sunrise, peak at noon, and decrease at sunset. The pain intensity of Spigelia and Sanguinaria changes with the sun. These two remedies have a slow onset and slow resolution of pain.
- Nighttime aggravation of pain is characteristic of Mercurius and Ferrum metallicum.
- Belladonna headaches are worse after 3:00 p.m.
- Thuja has two peaks of aggravation: 3 o'clock in the morning and 3 o'clock in the afternoon.
- Kali bichromicum headaches are worse between 3:00 a.m. and 5:00 a.m.
- Lachesis and Calcarea phosphorica headaches are worse upon waking in the morning, and Sulphur headaches tend to be aggravated around 11:00 a.m.

Case Management

Because each case is unique, I can give only general recommendations for case management. The following guidelines on potency, test dosing, and other topics can give you a general idea of homeopathic best practices, though the approach will vary for each individual patient.

Potency

If you are an inexperienced homeopath, start with small potencies. 6C would be a good place to begin. Give the remedy two or three times a day, under the tongue and on an empty stomach. If you are an experienced homeopath, you may choose the potency with which you are comfortable.

"Test Dose" Method

If a headache is present during my evaluation of a patient, I usually give a test dose right there in the office and check for a change of symptoms in 10 minutes. Despite the popular misconception that homeopathy acts slowly, you may see some improvement of the headache in 5-10 minutes if the choice of remedy is correct. So, after I give the remedy to the patient, I will either keep interviewing them or do something else in the office. Then in 10 minutes I come back and ask: "How is your headache?" And quite frequently, with a surprised expression, the patient tells me, "Oh, the headache is gone!" or "Oh, the headache is better!"

This "test dose" method, as I call it, is not conventional in homeopathy. I don't know any other homeopath who uses it. I introduced it in my practice after I started using a provocation-neutralization method for the diagnosis and treatment of food sensitivity. I found that a sequentially diluted (potentized) antigen cures an acute allergic reaction almost instantly.

The test dose method works best in cases with minimal organic pathology on the tissue level, such as headaches or muscle spasms. It helps me to develop a better understanding of the remedies.

Aggravation of Old Symptoms

When you start a homeopathic treatment, be aware of the possibility of a transient aggravation of old symptoms, which usually happens around day three. In the case of headaches, it may look like a migraine headache attack, for example. If that happens, it's actually a good sign and the patient should be aware of it.

So, when I give a homeopathic remedy to patients, I usually tell them that it may get worse before it gets better. If their symptoms become aggravated, it's usually short lasting, and I will ask the patient to stop taking the remedy. After the aggravation is over, they may start using the remedy on an as-needed basis, at the onset of another headache.

If the remedy was chosen correctly, patients usually report an increased energy level. If the patient reports a decreased energy level, you should stop the remedy, reevaluate the patient, and see if you can find a better simillimum.

Combining Homeopathy with Conventional Medications

Homeopathy does not interfere with conventional medications. There is no rush to discontinue a patient's headache medication, especially if it provides some relief. Keep in mind as well that some medications, such as benzodiazepines, cannot be discontinued abruptly.

If my patient is already taking a conventional medication, I don't stop it until we achieve a good result with the homeopathic remedy.

If a patient has been treated with multiple medications, he may not react even to the perfectly prescribed remedy. In this case, treatment with one dose of Sulphur 30C may help to restore the body's reactivity after suppression.

Combining Homeopathy with Neural Therapy or Trigger Point Injections

I frequently combine homeopathic treatment with neural therapy, which involves injecting a small amount of local anesthetic into certain points to clear the disturbances in the autonomic nervous system that underlie all illnesses and painful conditions. Both methods are powerful, and I try to discriminate between the effects of each method as thoroughly as possible. I often postpone homeopathic treatment until I have a chance to evaluate the effect of neural therapy on the patient for 24 hours.

If I perform a test dose of the homeopathic remedy in the office, I do it prior to administering neural therapy. I will then hold off on the next dose of the homeopathic remedy for 24 hours while I evaluate the effect of the neural therapy.

Trigger point injection (TPI) involves treating pain by injecting a small amount of local anesthetic into tender (hypersensitive) spots of tense muscle. TPI does not impose as many limitations on the combined use with homeopathy. However, test dosing should be performed prior to trigger point injections, and the patient may begin taking the homeopathic remedy a few hours after receiving the injections.

Trigger Foods, Food Sensitivity, & Diet

The significance of specific foods as headache triggers is vastly underappreciated and insufficiently studied. Doctors suggest nutritional modifications for the treatment of headaches infrequently and in a limited fashion. As a result, the impact of foods on health in general, and on triggering headaches in particular, is addressed nowadays primarily by alternative or holistic healers and laypeople. The medical community, for the most part, does not consider food sensitivity to be a valid subject for consideration.

We do know that food sensitivity and food intolerance involve different mechanisms from the classic, immune-mediated food allergy pathway—which is characterized by the development of Immunoglobulin E (IgE) antibodies reacting to food allergens.

The never-ending dispute over whether or not food sensitivity can be considered an allergy, or whether or not food sensitivity even exists, stems from the lack of consensus on which tests can be used to confirm it. The thinking goes, what cannot be reliably measured should not exist. This attitude is slowly changing because doctors are pressured by an increasing number of patients who feel that certain foods give them health problems.

In his 1810 *Organon of the Art of Healing*, the father of homeopathy, Samuel Hahnemann, emphasized that to remove obstacles to curing a condition or achieving permanent recovery, the physician must keep the patient on a diet of simple foods during treatment. This point is still valid today; however, the foods that we consume differ from those of Hahnemann's time due to various modifications and added chemicals. We ingest a lot of highly processed foods that are poisonous to the body, and one can make the case that some of these items should not even be classified as food. Toxins of all kinds can damage the intestinal microbiome and produce an additional strain on the immune system.

While any food can trigger headaches, wine and cheese are frequent culprits. Sulphates in wine are usually blamed for headaches, though if this is the case, drinking wines without preservatives should not cause headaches, and often they do. In many cases, wine triggers headaches for different reasons. Wine and certain cheeses are fermented foods made with the help of yeast. People who are sensitive to the Candida albicans yeast may react to wine, cheese, and other fermented foods like beer and bread. Candida is part of our normal intestinal flora; however, in cases of dysbiosis (microbial imbalance), patients become sensitive to it.

How do we develop a sensitivity to yeasts that are supposed to be a part of our normal intestinal flora? We can name many factors, but the widespread use of antibiotics and sugar are chief among them.

Gluten and milk (and milk products in general) are even more frequent triggers, but they can be difficult to trace as a cause of headaches. (By the way, one doesn't need to have celiac disease to be sensitive to gluten.) A few lucky people have headaches soon after consuming a trigger food, so the connection is clear. Unfortunately, most people develop a headache the next day or even a few days later, which makes it difficult to identify the trigger. Infrequent consumption of alcohol by migraine sufferers makes it easier to connect the headache with the wine they drank the night before. Yet daily consumption of gluten and milk products makes it more difficult to distinguish the impact of these foods on triggering headaches. We have a few special tests for food sensitivity, like provocation-neutralization and ALCAT, but they are costly and not always available.

An oral challenge feeding test is one test that we can easily do with the patient. First, they must stop eating the suspicious foods completely for 3–4 weeks and acknowledge a disappearance of headaches. To confirm this observation, they may re-introduce the food and carefully observe their health for the next three days. A return of headaches, fatigue, and other symptoms indicates sensitivity to this food.

Foods can trigger not only migraines but also tension headaches. And different types of headaches may be triggered by different foods in the same patient. I had a patient whose migraine headaches were triggered by milk, and tension headaches came on after eating eggs.

Why gluten and dairy? If you think our predecessors who ate them were just fine, think again. Humans have reported migraine headaches for thousands of years. Migraine headaches frequently run in families through generations.

Humans started consuming milk and wheat approximately 10,000 years ago with the domestication of cows and the introduction of farming. For millions of years before this period, they did not eat these foods. From an evolutionary standpoint, 10,000 years is too short a time to fully develop enzymatic mechanisms for processing these new foods. Ancient Jewish tradition, which goes back thousands of years, strictly regulated the consumption of dairy foods, apparently because Jews noticed early on that dairy is difficult to digest.

This is compounded by the fact that, in recent years, we've made many changes to the quality and composition of foods. Wheat today contains four times more gluten than it did in the past. We're also seeing changes to our intestinal flora due to the widespread use of antibiotics and toxic chemicals. Normal intestinal flora plays a huge role in digestion, and when we disrupt it our health suffers.

I give special consideration to coffee as a trigger of headaches. If you drink coffee occasionally, it is unlikely that it causes your headaches, unless you notice on a few occasions that your headaches start the same day or the day after you drink coffee. If you drink coffee to improve your mood and feel that your day will be ruined without it, don't fool yourself—you have a substance addiction. People are frequently sensitive to foods to which they are addicted. Headaches may be triggered not only by substance use but also by discontinuation. But you need to stop if you want to produce lasting improvements to your health.

For these important reasons, I often combine homeopathic treatment with nutritional modification to treat headaches. My minimal dietary recommendations for patients with headaches? Avoid gluten, dairy, alcohol, and foods with synthetic chemicals—at least during the time of treatment.

If you generally avoid dairy because you are sensitive to milk, but you inadvertently consumed food that contained it and developed a headache, you may take Lac defloratum (one dose of 30C), a homeopathic remedy made from cow's milk. For a similar situation in the case of gluten sensitivity, I use a homeopathic remedy made from wheat or, even better, from bread. Note that the treatment of food sensitivity symptoms is a vast topic that extends beyond the scope of this book. We may address it in greater detail in a future book.

May you be free from headaches in the meantime!

Index

P

R

S

About Doctor Ostrovsky

Igor Ostrovsky, MD, PhD, is currently in private practice in regenerative and integrative medicine in New York, NY. He focuses on systemic and local aspects of regenerative medicine, treating patients with homeopathy, neural therapy, acupuncture, prolotherapy, nutritional modification, and other modalities.

Dr. Ostrovsky has been using homeopathy in his medical practice for more than 20 years. He studied at the New York School of Homeopathy and went on to continue training with world-renowned homeopaths, including Bhawisha Joshi, MD (Hom) and Shachindra Joshi, MD (Hom).

In addition to being a member of the Homeopathic Medical Society of the State of New York, Dr. Ostrovsky is a founding member of the North American Academy of Neural Therapy, a charter fellow of the American College of Acupuncture, a fellow of the American Academy of Anti-Aging Medicine, and a diplomate of the American Academy of Integrative Pain Management.

Learn more about Dr. Ostrovsky at www.DoctorOstrovsky.com.

Made in United States
Orlando, FL
04 November 2026

90200101R00045